MW01264950

Pot Diet

How to Lose Weight with Marijuana

By

Jessica Lovett

*Copyright © 2018 – **CSBA Publishing House***

Published by:

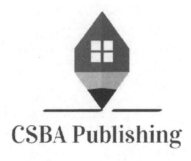

CSBA Publishing

CSBA Publishing House

Cover & Interior designed

By

Heather Ross

First Edition

DISCLAIMER

The author has made every effort to ensure that the information in this book is correct. However, it should be noted that the legal aspects of growing and consuming marijuana vary in different countries; readers are advised to use their own discretion and abide by the rules of their country for growing marijuana.

Also, this book is not intended to be a substitute for the medical advice of doctors. The reader is advised to consult a physician in matters relating to his/her health and weight loss before using this herb-based diet.

Any and all content provided here is for information only. The author is not claiming to cure any diseases, but strongly advises anyone suffering to seek proper medical attention.

Warning:

Marijuana, while becoming increasingly socially-acceptable, is not available in all states. Before starting this diet, check with your state to ensure that marijuana is legal. If you click on the following link, you'll discover the status of marijuana legalization state by state in the U.S.

http://www.governing.com/gov-data/state-marijuana-laws-map-medical-recreational.html

TABLE OF CONTENTS

INTRODUCTION

MARIJUANA AND MUNCHIES

The words come out of your mouth like a pair nearly unconsciously. Whether you've smoked marijuana for years or never touched the substance, the one thing everyone knows is that those who do smoke, get hungry. And society uses a catchy shorthand, "the munchies."

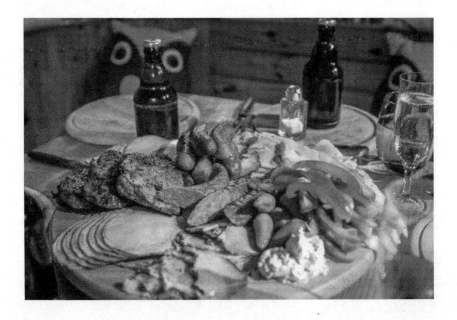

So, the following fact, printed in the esteemed *American Journal of Epidemiology*, that those who smoke weed on the average weighed less than the nonsmoker seems on the surface counterintuitive.

The study said that the obesity rates are about a third less for marijuana smokers.

As a pot smoker and a person who has tried just about every diet, I was quite surprised and more than a bit skeptical.

But that's not all; I read another article detailing a study, published in the *American Journal of Medicine* saying those who smoked cannabis, the scientific term for marijuana, regularly had a 15 percent lower fasting insulin rate, as well as a smaller waist. The size of the waistline, according to the medical community, is a direct correlation with a reduced risk of developing type II diabetes.

We'll go into the details of these studies in the next chapter, but for now, I want you to know how this research affected me.

What if you could take a habit that you already have, up until very recently, a bad habit, and turned it into an advantage and become one of those individuals who had a smaller risk of obesity as well as a lower insulin fasting rate?

Let me be clear on this: neither of these two studies said out rightly that if you smoked marijuana, you could lose weight. No, they stopped just short of that, but it didn't stop me from thinking about it.

The next thing I knew, I was doing more than just thinking about some wishful "what if" condition. I decided to see how much research was out there. I read just about everything I could find on the subject. I set out to see if it even was possible to lose weight, so I decided I had to change a few other bad habits as well. The first was a vow that I would have nothing but healthy food in the house. I decided to increase my exercise routine as well.

THE FIRST THIRTY POUNDS LOST

I began a marijuana and weight loss relationship without mentioning it to anybody. I guess I thought they would chastise me for smoking marijuana, which by the way, was legal in my state at the time of my experiment. If you decide to emulate the following simple steps, please check that marijuana has been legalized in your state.

Also, if you go to the gym after you've smoked, please handle all the equipment carefully. More often than not, if I had any doubt about my ability to exercise safely, I either didn't go or made sure I had a partner to go with me to keep an eye on my actions.

One more caveat: before you start any diet or exercise program, consult with your personal health care provider.

Below I reveal a quick outline of the routine of what I simply called "My Marijuana Diet." Again, remember I didn't tell anyone of my trial, for I knew that there would be more criticism, and I wanted to give this routine a fair try.

When I got home from work, I changed into my workout clothes before I had the opportunity to change my mind about going to the gym. Once dressed, I did my workout. Most days I went to the gym, but I have to confess that some days I stayed home and did a Pilates routine with or without a YouTube video, or a yoga workout.

Whichever one I chose, I made sure that I would then make a low-carbohydrate dinner. You'll notice at this point I haven't mentioned smoking any marijuana. That's because, at this point, I hadn't. Once I've made dinner and – here's the important part – before I ate, I smoked my pot.

The rest of the diet took care of itself, as you might expect. I waited for the munchies to hit – and boy, did they. I then went and ate dinner. And since I hadn't eaten supper yet, I scooped up my healthy meal because, quite frankly, I felt famished.

That's all there was to it. At least for the first 30 pounds.

At first, none of my friends and family noticed my weight loss. It wasn't until I hit that 30-pound mark that people began to make comments. Some asked me how I did it. The reactions ranged from laughter and disbelief (Yeah, right. I can understand if you don't want to share your secret) to those of veteran pot smokers who now saw their habit in a different light. More than one of my friends started the same routine

In the meantime, buoyed by my success, I've been doing even more research, and I'm discovering a whole host of facts about marijuana I never knew. What I learned wasn't restricted just to weight loss, though much of it was. But many of the facts I uncovered dealt with the benefits marijuana had on your physical body – regardless of your current health conditions.

What I mean is that if you're healthy now, smoking pot may help you keep certain disorders and diseases at bay. The more I learned, the more I incorporated as much of the new knowledge as possible into my dietary habits. Believe it or not, by the time I was done with my extensive research, I lost even more weight.

That's when, a voice here and a voice there, a family member, a co-worker or a friend told me I had to write a book about everything I learned and make public, what was, up until then, a very private diet.

The more I thought about it, the more I excited I got about the prospects. So I gathered everything I learned and brought it to you through this book. Depending on your view of marijuana, you may consider it nothing but trash or you may have an "aha" moment and give it a try. That's why, when I was writing, I decided that I would also talk about certain health benefits, many of which are directly related to the national obesity epidemic.

I've included in this book, in addition to a chapter on how to customize your own marijuana diet, a cannabinoid known by the initials of THCV. This substance is similar to the cannabinoid in the plant that provides you with a high, but it deals with your appetite. To be specific, it's known as an appetite suppressant.

While it seems incomprehensible, it's found in certain strains of marijuana. And I will show you how you can use this to help you lose weight.

MARIJUANA AND METABOLISM

One of the most exciting things I discovered about the health benefits of marijuana was recently reported through a Harvard health study. Marijuana can help you boost your metabolism. How many times have you been told or have discovered that your failed attempts to lose weight have more to do with your low metabolism, than your caloric intake or your sedentary lifestyle?

In fact, I found this news so exciting that not only did I include the latest research, but I talked a bit about the potential consequences of long-term low metabolism.

Some individuals discover that, regardless of what they do, they can't seem to lose weight. The persons find out that their weight problem is due more to harboring unresolved emotional issues as well as excess stressors. When one or more of these issues is resolved, you'll find you experience even more joy, peace of mind, and contentment than you ever thought possible.

CANNABIS AND CELIAC DISEASE

No discussion about the relationship between food and marijuana would be complete with a mention of celiac disease. A growing number of individuals are discovering that they are either intolerant to gluten, or suffer outright with the disease. These individuals are unable to eat grains with gluten, including bread and pasta. When they do, they suffer from stomach pains. For those with the disease, even just a bit of gluten can send their stomachs writhing with pain.

Who would have thought that smoking marijuana can help you manage this disease? It may not be a panacea to the growing disorder, but even if it lessens an accidental ingestion of gluten, it could be a godsend to some. I found it so amazing, that I devoted an entire chapter to it. I certainly hope you can find some relief in knowing this data.

Did you know that there are also strains of cannabis that can help you focus? Imagine using this strain to help you concentrate better while you're performing your exercise routine. It may very well be the one puzzle piece in your habits to kick start that weight loss regimen.

PUTTING IT ALL TOGETHER

This book is first and foremost a book dedicated to helping you discover ways in which you can use marijuana for your weight loss attempts. That's why there's a chapter in which I provide you with what I call a blueprint for losing weight with marijuana.

From my research – scientific studies and anecdotal evidence from others on the web – I've discovered that there is really any number of ways you can use marijuana to lose weight. From an appetite suppressant to a metabolism booster, and many other close-related topics, you can use marijuana to build your own program.

I'm giving you a starting point with this chapter. Use the parts of the blueprint you believe will be helpful to you and leave the rest. If you find you're not as successful as you'd like to be on your first try, then revisit the blueprint and try another route.

Don't become disappointed if you're not losing weight as quickly as you want. As you discover more about marijuana and weight loss, you'll find the right set of puzzle pieces and find that all the holes in your diet have been plugged.

But there's one more aspect in all of this that should give you hope: research on marijuana is still at its infancy. As more studies scrutinize the benefits of pot, there are bound to be even more benefits revealed along with ways to put the results into action.

In the meantime, follow me into Chapter 1, where we'll learn more about what pot has to do with weight loss as we dig deeper into the results of some of the latest scientific studies.

CHAPTER 1: WHAT DOES POT HAVE TO DO WITH WEIGHT LOSS

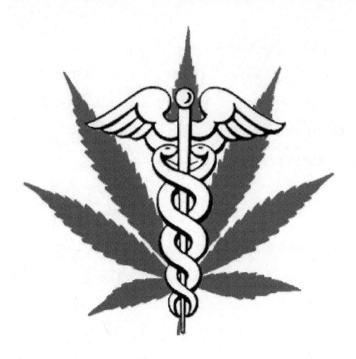

It's quite ironic that we talk about smoking marijuana in order to facilitate weight loss. After all, even those who have never smoked pot and know absolutely nothing about it – so they think – know that smoking pot causes a good case of the "munchies."

In other words, smoking marijuana increases your appetite. So how can it also be associated with weight loss?

Before we go into the various ways it could do just that, I want you to know I don't expect you to take my word for it. The way to start this discussion is by looking at just a few studies that have discovered these startling facts and statistics.

FACT #1

Those who smoke marijuana regularly – defined as three to four times a week – possess obesity rates that are about one third lower than the average person who doesn't smoke.

HOW DO WE KNOW THAT?

These numbers are the result of a study published in the 2011 issue of the *American Journal of Epidemiology*. Specifically, the scientific stats were garnered from research from two separate studies conducted in the United States. These studies involved 5,200 participants.

One of the studies demonstrated that 22 percent of nonsmokers were obese compared to only 14 percent of those who smoked pot.

The other study revealed similar results, with a full 25 percent of non-smoking individuals labeled obese. Of those who smoked pot daily, only 17 percent were classified as obese.

A similar study which compared the health of smokers and nonsmokers sparked intriguing results. In this study, the researchers looked at resting insulin rates.

FACT #2

Those who smoked marijuana had lower resting insulin rates, as opposed to those who didn't smoke. Those with higher insulin rates are at a greater risk of developing type II diabetes.

HOW DO WE KNOW THAT?

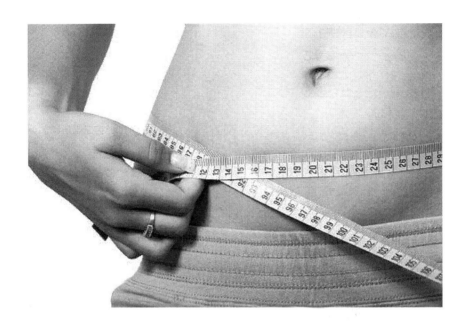

The results of this study were published in the *American Journal of Medicine.* The conclusion was that those who smoked marijuana approximately 3 to 5 times a week had resting insulin rates that were 16 percent lower than those who didn't smoke. In addition, they also had smaller waists. It's widely known in medical circles that the larger the waist size, the more at risk you're considered for this disorder.

HOW ARE WE TO INTERPRET THESE FACTS?

While these statistics are certainly intriguing, what exactly do they mean in relationship to marijuana and weight loss?

Scientists are quick to point out that these statistics are nothing more than an "association." Yes, there certainly is an interesting correlation between smoking marijuana, obesity rates, and even resting insulin rates. But they aren't ready to jump to any conclusions, especially the conclusion that smoking pot causes weight loss.

It's no secret that even the researchers themselves are, at least at the moment, left scratching their heads. But they're willing to propose several hypotheses to reconcile these seemingly disparate statistics.

THEORY NUMBER ONE: REPLACEMENT THEORY

In this supposition, scientists propose that marijuana smokers merely replace one habit for another. In this case, they replace overeating with smoking pot, and may not be taking in as many calories as it appears on the surface.

Here's the science behind the theory: eating what's known as "highly-palatable" foods that are not only high in fat and salt but also in refined sugar activates the reward center of your brain, called the nucleus accumbens. This alone gives you a type of "high." Researchers suggest that those who smoke marijuana are actually stimulating that same reward center, only minus the caloric intake.

THEORY NUMBER TWO

This hypothesis speculates on the use of medical marijuana. It's often used as an appetite stimulant, especially for AIDS patients or other disorders which dull your appetite.

In this theory, the researchers suggest that individuals in these studies may have been underweight at the time of the survey. Those suffering from these diseases are less likely to overeat than obese individuals with no health problems.

THEORY NUMBER THREE

Regular pot smokers become tolerant to their eating binges, so their bodies, therefore, aren't affected with a gain in weight.

They think that perhaps the cannabinoid receptor in the brain in charge of memory and appetite causes problems with their memories and trigger the munchies. However, as time goes by and marijuana smokers continue to smoke, these receptors are desensitized. This means the smokers are less likely to overeat, which in the long run prevents them from gaining weight.

OTHER HEALTH BENEFITS

While not directly related to weight loss, marijuana has other health benefits that deserve to be mentioned in this book. At the very least, these properties of marijuana are indicative of the new way society is looking at this drug. At most, it may be some benefit buried in this list (by no means all-inclusive) that could reveal clues as to why smokers may have a lower obesity rate and a reduced resting insulin level than nonsmokers.

It's difficult to get the point across on this topic or even show you the breadth of the capabilities of marijuana without looking, at least for a moment, at the large picture. Consider this a sneak peek. Perhaps someday researchers may be able to put all these diverse facts together and come up with a cohesive picture.

This is necessary because, believe it or not; marijuana contains more than 100 active components. One of these other ingredients in pot is a substance referred to simply as CBD, which refers to cannabidiol.

CBD is found abundantly in strains of pot used for medicinal purposes. On the other hand, these strands have little, if any THC, the substance that gives you the smoker's high and, in turn, the munchies.

RELIEF OF PAIN

Relieving pain is without a doubt the number one reason why medicinal marijuana is so widely used in this country. Granted, the plant's components are strong enough to quell the pain after major surgery or even a broken bone. That doesn't mean that individuals don't find relief with it for other, usually chronic, pain.

Part of the allure of this plant is that there is no fear of addiction, and it is far safer than dispensing strong pain-killing pharmaceuticals. Not only that, but it's impossible to overdose on medicinal marijuana. Because of this, you can also use it in place of Advil, Aleve, or other NSAIDs.

As a result, many individuals suffering from multiple sclerosis or generalized nerve pain find medicinal marijuana as a gift. And that's a good thing because, quite frankly, these folks have few other options aside from Neurontin, Lyrica, or opiates that have a sedative effect on their body.

MARIJUANA AS A MUSCLE RELAXANT

Many in the medical community believe that marijuana is one of the most effective muscle relaxants – bar none. Their patients agree nearly 100 percent, as testified by those who swear by its abilities. One of the best areas is that it's capable of actually slowing the rate of tremors in those who have Parkinson's disease.

In addition, it can also help with the following disorders: fibromyalgia, endometriosis, and interstitial cystitis, to name just a few.

MANAGING NAUSEA AND WEIGHT LOSS

Another common aspect of this is its ability to manage not only nausea and weight loss, but also in treating glaucoma, an eye condition that can lead to blindness.

CHAPTER 2: NOT ALL MARIJUANA IS CREATED EQUAL

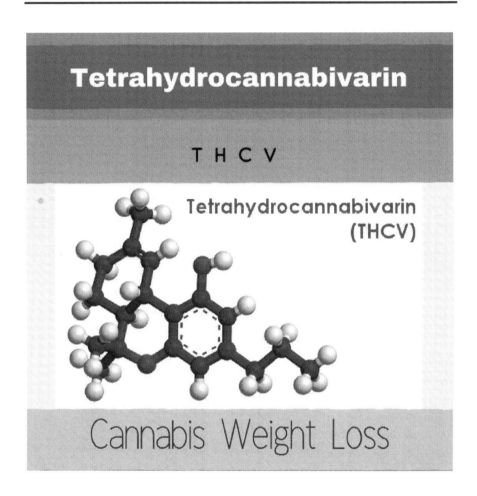

It's true. As we've seen in the previous chapter, we talked not only about the cannabinoid referred to simply by its initials, THC, but also those strains of the plant that contain CBD, which can be a near miracle for those dealing with pain and medical disorders of all kinds.

In this chapter, we're going to talk about a special strain of the plant that acts as an appetite suppressant. Yes, you read that right. An appetite suppressant.

The substance is closely related to THC, which gives the common strains of marijuana that have the ability to give you that high. It referred to THCV and could be another path you may want to consider in building your own personalized marijuana weight-loss program.

We've talked about THC, the compound that's in marijuana responsible for the high individuals receive when they smoke it. What's not quite so well-known is a similar compound, one called tetrahydrocannabivarin, or usually referred to as THCV.

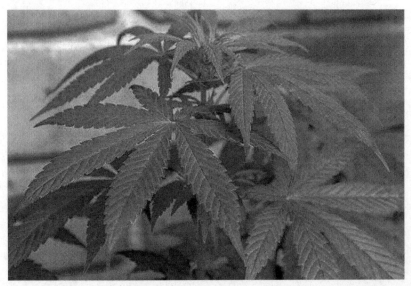

Ingesting THCV doesn't get you high, but that doesn't mean its effects are inert either. In fact, it's a quite amazing cannabinoid, quite unlike either THC or CBD, which gives marijuana its remarkable array of beneficial medical effects and more.

For our purposes, we're interested in its description as an appetite suppressant. This stands in contrast to THC, which may boost your appetite. While this may help the average consumer who would like to lose some weight, the medical community sends a warning to those individuals who are dealing with appetite loss or anorexia.

But more than that, THCV may help with other obesity-related disorders. In addition to functioning as an appetite suppressant, it also has the ability to battle diabetes. According to the latest scientific studies, THCV can help to regulate glucose levels, as well as reduce insulin resistance.

OTHER HEALTH BENEFITS

If you're plagued with panic attacks, this cannabinoid may help you overcome these – or at the very least reduce the number you have. It appears to work especially well for those who have been diagnosed with PTSD. And it does this without suppressing your emotions.

Believe it or not, THCV can actually help stimulate bone growth by promoting the production of new bone cells. Although it is not currently being used at the moment medically, this substance has garnered a lot of attention in this area. This makes scientists not only excited, but gives them hope for using it someday as an effective cure for osteoporosis.

Would you believe that this same substance has been well known to improve the memory of those with Alzheimer's? In the same way, THCV helps relieve tremors, motor control, and brain lesions. There is still much research being conducted in this area.

THCV: NOT IN ALL STRAINS OF MARIJUANA

Now that your appetite is whet, you're probably wondering where you can find strains of marijuana with the greatest amount of this appetite-suppressing cannabinoid. Most of the strains you may buy have trace amounts, if any, of it.

And the results are in . . .

At the moment, it appears that the strain called African sativa has the most abundant amount of THCV. This includes strains known as Landrace. This particular plant is native to not only Africa, but also Durban Poison. But there are other strains that also have this substance.

With the legalization of marijuana in many states, you can walk into "pot shops" and ask the assistants who work there what you're looking for and why. They'll be able to point you in the right direction.

GENETICS?

Yes, if you're experiencing difficulty finding a strain of African sativa, then you may have to trace their "ancestry", so to speak. Many types of marijuana have a hybridized African strain or two in their genetic background.

A plant, called Cherry Pie, may have high THCV levels if its "parent" is Durban Poison, one the plants it was mixed with. The sales assistants at your "pot shop" or dispensary can also help with this information. If not, you may want to visit a website called Leafly. Look at its strain pages.

If you're really serious about discovering if the marijuana you want has a high THCV content, you can ask at the location you buy it from to check lab-tested strains. Through this method, you can be ensured of a strain with an abundance of THCV.

The good news is that more and more marijuana will be bred with the purpose of increasing its THCV content.

While right now, you may have to hunt for it a bit, within a few years, you'll find that it will be in more strains in greater quantities. In the meantime, here are a few strains of marijuana that have among the highest quantity of this appetite suppressant.

6
HIGH THCV STRAINS
CANNABIS WEIGHT LOSS

1

DOUG'S VARIN

Doug's Varin is rare and trademarked. This is a strain that has been specially bred for no other reason but to increase its content of THCV.

2
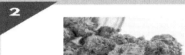

TANGIE

This strain is a hybrid sativa, the results of a strain of marijuana called Skunk and California Orange.

3

PINEAPPLE PURPS

Another sativa dominant type of marijuana, the Pineapple Purps are also bred with an eye to an abundant THCV content.

4

GIRL SCOUT COOKIES

It contains an abundant amount of THCV and has a taste that has been described as sweet as sugar.

5
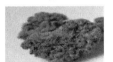

DURBAN POISON

Durban Poison is a South African landrace strain that produces high levels of THCV.

6
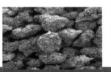

DUTCH TREAT

This strain of marijuana contains large resinous flowers in addition to its rich THCV content

DOUG'S VARIN

Doug's Varin is rare and trademarked. This is a strain that has been specially bred for no other reason but to produce a greater amount of THCV

Beyond that, you may enjoy its aromas of citrus and pine. No discussion of marijuana, even for weight loss, would be complete without mention of what kind of Effects you can expect from this strain. Once you smoke this, you may discover that you're energetic and clear-headed, free from any lingering anxiety.

TANGIE

This strain is a hybrid sativa, the result of a strain of marijuana called Skunk and California Orange. It'll provide you with a good amount of THCV as well as containing a distinguishing aroma and flavor. It's no secret why it's called "tangie." The taste and aroma are a blend between tangerines and oranges.

PINEAPPLE PURPS

Another sativa-dominant type of marijuana, the Pineapple Purps are also bred with an eye to an abundant THCV content. And yes, it's called pineapple because it has a flavor similar to that of sweet pineapple.

GIRL SCOUT COOKIES

Yes, this is definitely a strain of marijuana, as strange as it may sound. Again it contains an abundant amount of THCV and has a taste that has been described as sweet as sugar. This is, no doubt, the origin of its name.

DURBAN POISON

Durban Poison is a South African landrace strain that produces high levels of THCV. The large resin glands on the dense, chunky flowers offer a sweet, earthy flavor of pine and a euphoric, energizing cerebral experience.

DUTCH TREAT

This strain of marijuana contains large resinous flowers in addition to its rich THCV content, if you like earthy flavors of fruit as well as eucalyptus and pine. Other benefits of Dutch Treat include stress relief and a euphoric feeling.

CHAPTER 3: MARIJUANA AND METABOLISM

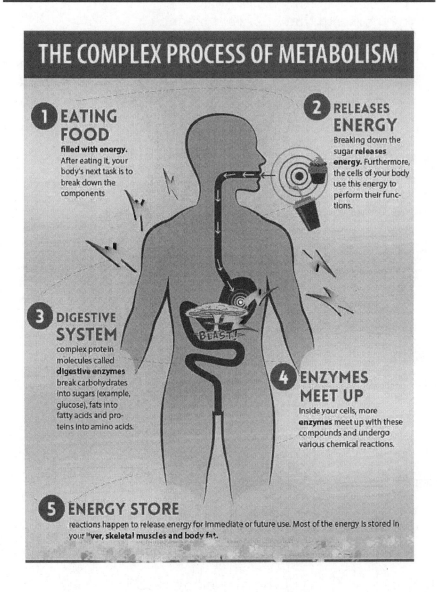

THE COMPLEX PROCESS OF METABOLISM

1 EATING FOOD filled with energy. After eating it, your body's next task is to break down the components

2 RELEASES ENERGY Breaking down the sugar releases energy. Furthermore, the cells of your body use this energy to perform their functions.

3 DIGESTIVE SYSTEM complex protein molecules called digestive enzymes break carbohydrates into sugars (example, glucose), fats into fatty acids and proteins into amino acids.

4 ENZYMES MEET UP Inside your cells, more enzymes meet up with these compounds and undergo various chemical reactions.

5 ENERGY STORE reactions happen to release energy for immediate or future use. Most of the energy is stored in your liver, skeletal muscles and body fat.

The latest research shows, according to some studies, that marijuana can increase your metabolism. This is good to know when you're incorporating smoking marijuana in your weight loss program. In a nutshell, this fact suggests that simply smoking marijuana alone may actually make it easier for those pounds to drop off.

But it also bodes well for at least a potential protection from the burgeoning disorder called Metabolic X, a combination of approximately three benchmarks which may make you a prime candidate for diabetes.

If you've been told that you may have difficulty losing weight because your metabolism is slow, you're not alone.

Of course, knowing that there are others with slow metabolisms doesn't do a thing to increase yours. Imagine my surprise when I discovered that marijuana could play an amazing role in affecting the metabolism rate. Certain types of marijuana can increase your metabolism and keep the symptoms and benchmarks usually associated with Metabolic X Syndrome at bay.

The problem is when people tell you that, they usually don't tell you what steps you can follow to boost your metabolism so that you can burn calories faster. That's how it was for me, at least. More than one of my friends voluntarily "diagnosed" me. It's as if, when they would inform me, my metabolism would magically increase.

In the simplest sense, one's metabolism involves your body's set of chemical reactions that are needed for the development of your normal growth and development. All of your actions are fueled by energy. The catch to this is that you need to take it in from the outside environment, then convert it into a form your body can use.

There are only a few ways in which this can be done. Eating for energy, without a doubt, is the most important way you can achieve this goal. So, in other words, you can describe metabolism as digestion and the reactions that the digestion triggers. The easiest way to explain it, is: convert the food you eat into fuel to run your bodily functions and sustain your life.

Metabolism refers to the process of the conversion itself. The speed at which this process occurs is called your basal metabolic rate, most of the time simply referred to by its initials, BMR.

How does all of this Affect your Weight?

Once you understand what metabolism is, then it becomes easier to understand its relationship to your weight. If you need to speed your slow metabolism, what you need to do is eat a healthier diet and build muscle. Let's face it, it's nothing you haven't heard before. The problem is that when you don't have the energy to take this advice – building muscle – you run smack dab into a vicious circle; you can't exercise without energy, and you can't acquire much more energy without exercise.

That's where the beauty of using marijuana to increase your metabolism may come in. But before we go there, let's take this strand of discussion one or two steps farther. What could potentially occur to your health if you're not able to boost your metabolism to lift yourself out of that "slow metabolism" rut?

Five Risk Symptoms

Some of the many problems involved in a slow metabolism involve the long-term effects. If you continue to accept the fact that you have a slow metabolism without challenging it, you are opening yourself up to eventual unhealthy consequences. Among some the more disturbing disorders and diseases, you're at an increased risk for heart disease, diabetes, high blood pressure, and high cholesterol levels.

In fact, you set yourself up for developing the syndrome – a series of five benchmark symptoms – that could raise your chances of risk. To be exact, the five symptoms are listed below:

1. *Increased blood pressure defined as 130/85 mmHg.*
2. *Insulin resistance as exemplified by high blood sugar levels.*
3. *Excessive fat around your waistline.*
4. *High triglyceride levels.*
5. *Low levels of the "good" type of cholesterol.*

If you have just one of these factors, it doesn't mean that you have the metabolic syndrome. But possessing just one of these symptoms does increase your odds of eventually developing heart disease. However, if you have three or more of these symptoms, it indicates you already have the Metabolic X Syndrome. What does that mean? It doesn't mean you're going to develop Diabetes II, but it certainly is an indication that your risk of health complications is much greater than those without those disorders.

The bottom line is, the Metabolic X Syndrome is an accurate harbinger about your ultimate chances of developing obesity. When it comes to this problem, the two most important risk factors, according to some medical specialists, are central obesity or excessive fat around the middle and the upper areas of your body.

The second risk factor is that of insulin resistance. This means that your body is having difficulty using glucose. The factors of Metabolic X Syndrome, as serious as they can be at heightening your risk of not only diabetes but other degenerative disorders and diseases, are not the only risk factors.

Your odds of developing this disorder increase with age, if you have a family history of metabolic syndrome, and leading a sedentary life. Another deciding factor is that women are at a greater risk if they have been diagnosed with polycystic ovary syndrome.

If you do develop this syndrome, you may eventually find there are complications that may emerge. These complications include hardening of the arteries, better known as atherosclerosis, heart attack, kidney disease, stroke, nonalcoholic fatty liver disease, peripheral artery disease, as well as cardiovascular diseases.

And of course, you are definitely increasing your chances of developing type II diabetes. And if you believe that you'll be able to control it with pills or even injections, you better think again.

The longer you have diabetes, the greater your odds of developing these complications: retinopathy, or damage to your eyes, and neuropathy, or nerve damage with eventual amputation of your limbs.

So, being diagnosed with diabetes really is serious.

ENTER THE USE OF MARIJUANA

The really stunning notion of all of this is that smoking marijuana has the potential to help you avoid these illnesses and symptoms.

The irony is that some researchers have known about the remarkable powers of marijuana over your metabolism for almost have a century. It's true. A 1978 study published in the *American Review on Respiratory Diseases* studied the metabolism as well as the breathing of eight individuals. It was revealed that those who smoked marijuana all had faster metabolic rates than those who didn't.

The research has been revived by a Harvard Medical School professor of medicine who found similar results. He concluded that those who smoked processed carbohydrates more efficiently than nonsmokers.

But that's not all. Smokers had lower fasting insulin levels than nonsmokers. And yes, the smokers also maintained smaller waists, another prevented potential symptom of Metabolic X Syndrome.

This study has also been replicated and published in the medical journal *Obesity*, which stated that marijuana use was "statistically associated with lower body mass, as well as a lower fasting insulin level."

That's only a part of the story, though. The best is yet to come. Those who used marijuana not only had lower obesity rates than nonsmokers, but they also possessed the lowest rate of obesity and body mass index.

CHAPTER 4: MARIJUANA AND EMOTIONAL EATING AND STRESS

Good Morning Let the Stress Begin...

Many times, individuals have a difficult time losing weight because the cause of their being overweight in the first place is emotions and/or stress.

Which one of us hasn't been in this position? After a long, stressful day at work, you come home, sit down, and then it happens. You head for the kitchen cabinets searching for that leftover bag of potato chips, Doritos, or even a handful of cheese puffs.

But wait, you and millions of others like you go through this ritual after you've already hit the vending machines at work, including a candy bar here, a bag of pretzels there, and... well, we need not go much farther.

Or perhaps you head straight for the freezer toward that quart of ice cream.

Stress. Chronic stress.

It isn't surprising that, as a society, we try to "eat our way to stress relief." And while we haven't been totally successful at managing stress in this fashion, we do have something to show for our efforts. The majority of adults are either overweight or obese.

If that's the only result we get from our poor attempts at managing stress, you can say with confidence this method is not working very well for us. Not only do we tend to overeat under stress, but we tend to overeat with unhealthy foods.

Take a look at these amazing statistics. You can be sure that within a month – a 30 day-period of time – approximately 38 percent of adults have overeaten and have done so on unhealthy foods to self-manage their chronic stress. Half of these adults, nearly 50 percent, admit to "stress eating" several times a week.

Why do we do it? The answers are simple; it distracts them from the stress. At least, that's what 33 percent of those who eat under stress confess to. Another 27 percent also admit to eating as a way to actually manage their stressful feelings, and another 34 percent confess they do it purely out of habit.

Those are compelling statistics but take a deep breath; there are still a few more numbers to take into consideration when it comes to food and stress. In a 30-day period, 30 percent of Americans have confessed to actually skipping a meal, and they admit doing this at least once a week.

Of those who skip at least one meal a day because of their stressful days, 67 percent simply say they aren't hungry. Another 26 percent explained they didn't have the time to eat.
So how do they feel about their ability to manage stress intelligently after all this?

Needless to say, not many of these folks think it solved their problems. In fact, nearly half of them – 49 percent – say they feel disappointed in themselves. Another 46 say they feel "bad" about their bodies, and 36 percent of them describe themselves as feeling sluggish at best and lazy at worst. The final statistic is that out of those who skip meals, 22 percent say they end up irritable.

SHORT-TERM VERSUS LONG-TERM STRESS

When you're subjected to short-term, or acute stress, you may discover that your body reacts differently. Many individuals faced with a single stressful incident, and not the daily grind type of stress, discover that their body reacts by shutting down their appetite. Several sections of the brain work together with the adrenal glands to quell your desire to eat.

If the stress continues and inevitably transforms itself into long-term, chronic stress, then the body starts working differently. In this situation, your adrenal glands release another hormone that may stimulate your appetite. Specific hormone levels should fall, but if the stress persists, this may not subside. Instead, it stays at that high alert level. At times, even if the stress does subside, your hormone levels may get "stuck," and your appetite doesn't return to normal right away.

MORE THAN RANDOM CHOICES: FATS AND SUGAR

You noticed at the beginning of those statistics we cited some of the foods people most often choose when stressed out – those laden in fat and sugar. This preference is not just a random choice on their part, even though they believe it might be. Many scientific studies have shown that when we undergo either physical or emotional distress, our intake of foods are rich in fat, sugar, or both.

Those high hormone levels we spoke about earlier combined with elevated insulin levels are responsible for this reaction. At least that's what scientists believe at the moment.

Regardless of the reason, the bottom line is that you're basically faced with an appetite that is out of control. But, amazingly, once you begin to munch on these high fat or sugar foods, your appetite slowly begins to transform. It's as if the food "tames" that wild appetite. That is that these types of foods actually help control the activity of the brain that produces the stress, along with the emotions that tag along behind it.

These foods, which we have nicknamed "comfort" foods, really are just that. Specialists now speculate that these foods are a great contributor to that relief.

Research conducted at Harvard University has revealed that this chronic stress, combined with other problems, is associated with weight gain. But if that's true, scientists needed to discover if those test subjects already carried that excess weight at the beginning of the study.

That means, in the working world, that if you enter a chronically stressful situation already carrying excess pounds, by the time the stress slows down, you're likely to have gained weight. That's not necessarily so for those who enter the same circumstances at their target weight.

Before we talk about how the use of marijuana may help you to lose weight, let's up to the health ante here. While weight gain is one thing, it's the long-term consequences of that weight on your health that's really worrisome. Make no mistake about it – chronic stress can claim your good health and turn it around quicker than you can imagine.

Believe it or not, there are three basic types of stress, or as some scientists call them, "channels" in which your body can be affected by the stress. They are called environmental, bodily, and emotional.

Environmental stress is the kind that comes from your surroundings. Imagine walking down a city street and coming across a construction site. The sound of a jackhammer is so loud that it startles you and cuts into your concentration. Now, that's environmental stress. Pollution, which affects your body, is also another excellent illustration of this type of stress.

The second type of stress is the kind that is channeled through your body – that is, illness, sleep deprivation, and even poor eating habits.

Emotional stress varies from the other two because it's essentially triggered by how you interpret your life and other events. This one is a bit more complex to understand without an example.

Let's say that you have a colleague at work who is passive-aggressive. You may choose how to react to him, but this may be considered emotional stress if you take his actions personally. If you don't take his behavior as a personal slap against you, then the amount of stress you acquire from this is far lower.

FIVE WAYS YOUR BODY REACTS TO STRESS

Below are just a few quick ways how your body reacts to this kind of stress.

YOUR BODY AGES FASTER

The cells of your body and your organs begin to slow and are not operating at their full potential

BUILD-UP OF SUGAR

Originally, in our evolution, the sugar that is released when we meet stress was used to prepare us for what's been called the fight or flight response. For our ancestors, it was either fight whatever was facing them – for our hunter-gatherer ancestors, it was usually a large mammal – or turn around and run with all of their might (flight).

Either way, your body puts the sugar to good use. Today, the same reaction occurs. Stress signals to your body that sugar needs to be released. But if we can neither run nor fight the stress, our body doesn't use that sugar. Instead, your body stores it as fat.

YOUR BLOOD THICKENS

You may wonder about why this occurs, since it's not quite as obvious as the other two. The thickening of your blood allows your blood to carry more oxygen throughout your body.

Again, this is your body preparing for the fight or flight response. When your body doesn't use either of these options, the blood has no place to go but to build up what's referred to as "plaque" on the walls of your arteries.

DEPRESSES THE IMMUNE SYSTEM

This bodily reaction is probably something you're far more familiar with. I'm sure you've noticed when you're stressed for any reason, it appears your chances of getting a cold or flu are heightened. No, it isn't your imagination.

CHANCES OF DEVELOPING OTHER DISEASES

Chronic stress can make any disorder or disease you already have worse. Stress has been linked to health problems such as Parkinson's disease, multiple sclerosis, as well as heart disease and diabetes.

You're now beginning to understand how vital it is that you learn how to manage stress intelligently. Yes, there are plenty of prescription drugs on the market that you can take. But many of these carry adverse side effects. A growing number of persons are having second thoughts about using pills for stress and anxiety. Meditation is also more popular than ever to rein in your body's response.

You may be wondering how to employ this information so you can incorporate marijuana – and the proper type of strain – into your weight loss efforts. This may be a particularly vital issue if you believe part of your excessive weight is due to your natural reaction to stress, which is to eat foods containing a large amount of fat and sugars.

Scientific studies on marijuana are in their infancy, so finding anything greater than anecdotal evidence that it can actually help you respond to stress is difficult. That's why a study from Washington State University is exciting. It confirms that smoking marijuana can help you manage your response to stressors better. Specifically, researchers concluded that there was no discernable difference in those individuals who smoked marijuana to either psychological or physiological stress, than a non-stressed circumstance. Those who did not use marijuana were subjected to the same simulated stressful circumstances, and had a much higher level of cortisol.

Some parts of the study are interesting, so they deserve a bit of attention on our part.

Let's talk about the "stress" the researchers put the participants through. The researchers divided the participants into two groups. 40 of these individuals were identified as regular marijuana smokers, and 42 others were considered nonusers. Members of each group were asked not to smoke marijuana on the day of testing.

At the beginning, all participants underwent the same test to discover their stress level. Individuals were randomly chosen to undergo either the "no-stress" version of the test or the "high-stress" version.

During the no-stress test, participants placed a hand in a dish of lukewarm water for a minimum of 45 seconds and no longer than 90 seconds. In addition, they were requested to count from 1 to 25.

For the high-stress case study, individuals were instructed to place one hand in ice-cold water for 45 to 90 seconds. Additionally, they were also asked to count backwards from 2,043 (yes, you read that right) by groups of 17. Then, when they made a mistake, they were given "negative feedback."

But wait, the "stress" doesn't end there. Test subjects were also monitored by a web camera, which was displayed directly in front of the participant.

Stress levels were again taken at the end of the simulation. The research indicates that smoking marijuana may make you more resilient in dealing with stress. Those who regularly smoked marijuana had consistently lower stress levels regardless of the group they were in.

If you think that you may be able to handle stress better and eat less high-fat and sugar-loaded foods during stressful situations, you may very well want to incorporate marijuana purposely to do just that.

Having said that, the last question you're probably asking yourself is: What strains of the plant would work the best?

Strain of Marijuana	Description
Cannatonic	The active ingredient in marijuana that can help relieve stress is CBD, which gives you that calm feeling without any psychoactive effects.
Green Crack	Though it's best known for increasing your energy, as a sativa strain it can provide mental clarity while calming you without any side effects of drowsiness or lethargy.
Grape God	A hybrid strain, it's the offspring of God Bud and Grape God. You need to know that this is a potent strain, so if you decide to use it, expect long-lasting effects. Stress can make you depressed, many assert, so the effects of this strain

	are to make you joyful. And let's face it, it's hard to worry when you're feeling good.
Blue Dream	It's a hybrid with a sativa-dominant nature. You'll love the fact that it provides you with a whole body feeling of relaxation and calm. The catch to this strain is that it contains a higher than average THC level than the other strains listed here. That means you'll receive a higher than average "high" from this plant as well.
Super Silver Haze	This strain, too, is a hybrid. It's the result of a union with Skunk, Northern Lights, and Haze. It works at relieving stress, according to those who have used it, a "full-body" high, while at the same time boosting your energy. As you know, one of the effects of stress is to steal your energy.
AK-47	Though you couldn't tell this by its name, this strain does a great job of making you "mellow", and at the same time helping you to focus and be more

> aware of your surroundings. This allows you, in essence, to focus on something other than what's stressing you out.

Know that there are strains of marijuana that relieve stress and, in turn, help you to resist reaching for that quart of ice cream, the bag of chips, or the candy bar. There's no "proper" way to use these strains. You may not only want to try a variety of strains to see which works best for you, but you may also want to decide the most effective way to use them.

This may not happen overnight, but it you put a bit of effort into it, you'll discover the perfect balance between managing stress and marijuana's role in this process.

In the next chapter, we'll talk about how some strains of marijuana may help you lose weight by reducing your body's reaction to gluten. This is the perfect chapter not only for those who have been diagnosed with Celiac Disease, but also for those individuals who believe they may have an intolerance to the substance found in a wide array of our frequently used grains.

CHAPTER 5: CANNABIS AND CELIAC DISEASE

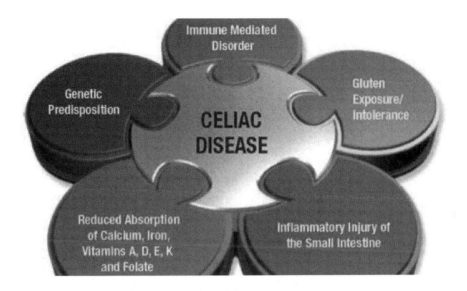

Are you having a difficult time dropping that last 20 pounds or so on your diet? Are you upset because the last several pounds are in the stomach area and there doesn't seem to be anything you can do to flatten your belly?

What if I told you that the last 20 pounds aren't due to your overeating or even your lack of exercise? Instead, consider that perhaps at least of a portion of that weight could be what's been labeled a "wheat belly."

The first time this term was used with any consistency was in a natural health book called *Wheat Belly,* by William Davis. He argues, quite convincingly, that the small belly many of us carry around is actually due to difficulty in digesting wheat and other grains because of their gluten content.

Believe it or not, the marijuana diet can help you lose those last 20 or so pounds, not only by revving up your metabolism, but by actually healing some of the damage done by years of consuming gluten. The inability to digest gluten is called celiac disease.

Before you skip this chapter because you're sure you don't suffer from this disorder, consider just the following two facts:

Statistics show that only approximately one in 133 Americans are plagued with this disorder. That's about one percent of the population, which doesn't seem like many. However, that's only one side of the coin. While one percent may be formally diagnosed with this painful disorder, there are many more individuals who have varying degrees of intolerance to gluten.

These people find that they feel much better overall when they stay away from products containing gluten.

Approximately 83 percent of individuals with celiac disease have gone undiagnosed or have been misdiagnosed with other disorders.

So, what is Celiac Disease?

Celiac disease is a disorder of the small intestine which causes damaging, sometimes very painful digestive problems. Those who have this condition have found they are unable to eat wheat, barley, and rye. If that weren't bad enough, this disorder could also block many of the nutrients your body requires from reaching their proper destinations.

If you have a clear case of celiac disease, there's no need telling you what the symptoms are. You're all too familiar with the pain. Yet the amazing fact about the symptoms is the varying signs from one individual to another. The most common signs that may indicate you have celiac disease include diarrhea, fatigue, and weight loss.

But those aren't the only symptoms. Others include bloating and gas, abdominal pain, nausea, vomiting, and even constipation.

The most surprising symptoms, however, seem to have nothing to do directly with the disease, which could very well be the reason it's so often misdiagnosed.

A wide range of possible symptoms of celiac disease are listed in the table below.

A Few of the Symptoms of Celiac Disease

Anemia	Osteoporosis	Osteomalacia
Dental enamel damage.	Mouth ulcers.	Headaches.
Fatigue.	Damage to the nervous system, displayed in numbness and tingling in the feet and hands, problems with	Cognitive impairment.

	balance.	
Joint pain.	Hyposplenism, or reduced functioning of the spleen.	Acid reflux.
Heartburn.	Foggy mind.	

This is all interesting you may say, but what does this have to do with marijuana – and especially my losing weight with the help of the plant? Much more than you may realize, thanks to a unique set of factors.

The best part of this relationship is that it's been confirmed by scientific research. The most telling of the studies conducted in Italy biopsied the small intestines from those diagnosed with the disorder. The researchers specifically examined the body's natural cannabinoid receptors. They play a vital part in controlling inflammation and dysfunction of the intestines.

The results of this action showed that those individuals with the active disease possessed more receptors than those who had been treating it with a minimum of a gluten-free diet.

In the following chapter, we're going to pull it all together and give you some ideas of how to construct your own personalized weight loss diet with the aid of marijuana.

CHAPTER 6: A BLUEPRINT OF HOW MARIJUANA CAN AID IN WEIGHT LOSS

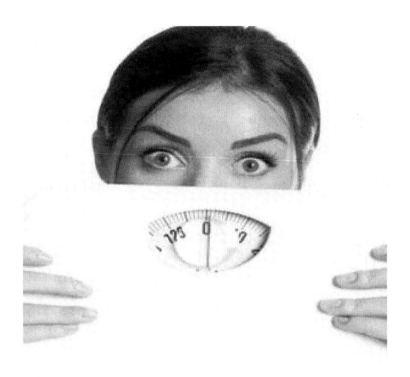

Marijuana has never been a more popular weight-loss aid. No doubt at least part of the credit is due to the fact that the plant is now legal in so many states.

Though it has an infamous reputation for kick-starting your appetite, nearly everyone who has ever smoked it has commented on the cravings they've developed. Casually called "the munchies," it's a stereotype of the effects of using it.

At the same time, though, we've learned that those who smoke this drug are less obese than the average person. It only makes sense that individuals – and especially scientists – would not only be asking why, but also wonder if there is a way you can use it to aid in an effective weight loss program.

As we've presumed all along in this book, there is a resounding yes. With a few – and I mean very few – changes in some of your habits, you may have one of the most effective aids in losing weight.

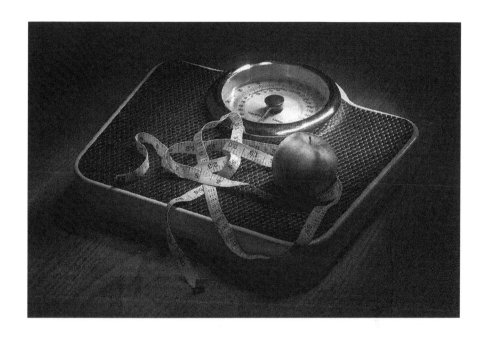

DEFINE YOUR GOALS

The first step of any diet is determining what you want to accomplish. If you jump into any diets without a plan and an intent, two things are likely to occur. The first is that you may become disappointed and quit because you can't track your success. The second is that you may stay with it for a time, but you may not see any type of progress simply because you've failed to state what you want out of it.

Do you want to increase stamina?
How much weight do you wish to lose?
What areas of your body do you wish to target?

Knowing this will make your dieting easier. Once you've set your goals, check out the factors that will make your efforts a success.

Use the appropriate strains of pot

Whatever your goal is, checking out what strain of marijuana would provide you with the biggest boost in this area is always a wise decision.

Munchies?

When the munchies hit, be prepared with some healthy foods. This may sound like a tall order. Indeed, you may not be able to do this overnight. The point of the goal, though, is to move at your own speed from junk food to healthier food. Take your time transitioning your eating habits. If you force healthy foods before your body's ready, it will only end in one result: Backsliding to those junk foods.

Juicing

Juicing? Sure, it's a great way to get the vitamins and minerals your body requires in large amounts that can help you with your exercise program.

Continue your exercise routine

Whatever you do, don't stop exercising. It's essential for any plan for losing weight, but it is especially important to this diet. The combination of exercise and the right strain of pot for you can enhance your efforts. There is more information on this later in this chapter.

Overall, make healthier food choices

Take that effort you're putting into making your marijuana munchies healthier, and continue applying those actions to your entire diet. Don't try to change everything you eat overnight. Make one or two changes at a time and don't add any more until you've got the first couple in your diet routine.

Reduce stress

Of course, if you do the other suggestions above, you'll be better prepared to handle the stresses that are handed to you. But beyond that, evaluate your life and try to eliminate stress in any way you can. You may want to put less pressure on the importance of your work, maybe even start searching for another job that appears to be less stressful.

FIVE-STEP PLAN TO SEE WILD SUCCESS IN MARIJUANA DIET

Now, that you know what's expected of you to make the marijuana diet a wild success, here are the basic steps of the plan.

1. Use marijuana.

I thought I'd start with the easiest first. Before you start, be prepared. That may mean that you'll have to go to your local marijuana dispensary to purchase a strand that is intended to motivate and energize you, while at the same time will reduce your appetite, even if only slightly.

2. Stock your refrigerator with healthy foods.

Make sure you have some healthy foods in the house so you will at least have a better choice available.

3. Exercise.

Now is the time to start a dedicated exercise program. You may visit the gym, go jogging, bicycling, or dive into yoga or Pilates. The idea is to do what interests you so you aren't tempted to just walk away from it. Be sure to smoke a bit of weed, some experts say no more than three puffs, before you perform your chosen activities. Then, either during a break in your activity or after you're done, you do your munching on some healthy snacks.

4. Drink plenty of liquids

Just make sure they aren't alcoholic drinks. There are several reasons for this, not the least of which is that drinking alcohol contributes to weight gain. Instead, you'll want to reach for water, and beyond that, some encourage consuming raw cannabis leaf juice.

Take only the green leaves of the plant and put them in a juicer. Yes, you'll probably need a good amount of leaves, but those individuals who have done this are enthusiastic about it. Some users even call it "nature's magic cure-all juice." One hint, drink a glass of water both before you drink the pot juice, as well as after you drink it.

5. Make the program part of your lifestyle.

Don't make your marijuana intake and subsequent exercise an isolated part of your day. Make it, instead, only a small part of a well-rounded, healthy lifestyle. What do I mean by this?

When you get home from work or your workout, be sure you de-stress. You may want to smoke more marijuana, or you may want to spend some time meditating. Whatever you do, be sure that you prepare a healthy meal. If you're craving pizza for dinner, the toppings should be as healthy as possible.

"Going healthy" means staying away as much as possible from refined flour, processed foods, and simple carbohydrates like refined sugar. Instead, make your meals out of whole grains, vegetables, fruits, as well as meat and seafood.

This chapter only presents a broad outline of how you can incorporate marijuana into your efforts. Keep in mind that these aren't the only portions of the "diet" you need; you'll still need to use a standard weight loss program. If you have one has worked for you in the past, then you have an advantage.

How much do you smoke?

If you plan on smoking marijuana prior to your workout, then you should be smoking a lot less than if you just want to get that recreational high. This is vital, since depending on your plans, you may be operating with weights, a treadmill, or a stationary bicycle.

EXERCISE: THE FOUNDATION OF ANY GOOD WEIGHT-LOSS PROGRAM

For those of you who thought you were getting off scot-free from any exercise requirement, I hate to be the bearer of bad news. It's hands down, the best way to lose weight.

And when you combine it with various strains of marijuana to boost the exercise potential, the results are even better.

But before we talk about the optimum strains to smoke for optimum results, it's essential you know how this plant affects you. Of course, you want to know how to make the most out of your exercise time. But you also want to be sure that you don't put yourself or anyone around you in danger.

First off, if you feel any doubt about how high you are and plan on going to the gym, you're probably too high to go. Another option would be to grab a friend to keep an eye on you. It may sound childish, but it's much better to be careful.

The other factor you may not realize is that before you run off to exercise, you don't need to smoke as you do on a recreational level. Simply one or two puffs on a cigarette can give you just about the perfect amount of the substances. This should provide you with a mild high while giving you the other effects (depending on the strain you've chosen) to make a positive change in your workout.

You don't want to smoke too much before exercising, only to find that you've crashed, filled with fatigue and lethargy before you've even finished it. Only you can find the amount that's good for you. As you're well aware, everyone has a different reaction to marijuana. Once you find your "sweet spot" of a high that also gives you that exercise experience you crave, stay with it. You've found something remarkable.

YOU'VE NEVER SMOKED POT BEFORE?

Smoking then immediately exercising might not be the best way to begin either a smoking routine or an exercise program. If you're seriously considering smoking just try out this diet, then you'll need to do some pre-exercise smoking. You may want to take a week or more to test out the effect it has on you.

MARIJUANA AND PAIN

We've mentioned there are certain strains containing substances that are excellent at reducing pain. If your goal in exercising is to perform more repetitions, attain more stamina for your jogging program, or just going that extra mile or two on that treadmill, give these strains some thought.

If you're already in a serious exercise plan, then you know how tough those last couple of repetitions or that final mile can be. If you smoke the proper strain, you may be able to reduce the pain associated with that.

MARIJUANA AND FOCUS

When you perform your favorite physical activities, one of the best feelings is getting in the zone or the flow. This takes place when you feel energized, and become hyper-aware of not only your body, but your environment as well. Everything around you looks brighter.

Of course, you don't need marijuana to get into this zone, but it becomes easier when you smoke the proper strain. This has benefits, by the way, outside of an exercise program. We've talked about this in the chapter about managing stress intelligently.

Many individuals experience this by doing what's referred to as micro-dosing. But providing your body with even a small amount of marijuana, you will find that an increase in your focus could help you refine your program. You may use it to do another repetition or to concentrate more on your form if you're weight lifting, or perfecting your backhand if you're playing tennis.

Marijuana contains various cannabinoids and terpenes, substances that are capable of boosting your energy level, increasing your focus, minimizing pain, and shortening your recovery period following your exercise. It has everything you need to jumpstart your efforts.

In addition to that, your body has its own endocannabinoid system, and believe it or not, smoking marijuana can be a valuable aid in keeping this system well-balanced.

I won't bog you down with all the scientific details; you can research them later if you like. But I'd like to use an analogy. It's simple, but it makes a great illustration. For a moment, think of your body being made of two large puzzles. The first puzzle is your brain as well as your nervous system. The second puzzle is the rest of your body. This is your endocannabinoid system.

The truth of these two puzzles is that they are seldom – if ever fully – put together, there's always a piece missing here, or a piece we need to fill in there. The missing pieces are what scientists refer to as cannabinoid receptors, or simply CB receptors.

For our purposes, we're considering CB1, located in your head and central nervous system. CB2 is found throughout parts of your body. Our brains are called endocannabinoids. Conveniently, they are able to fill in any of the empty spaces.
The phytocannabinoids, those found in marijuana, can also fill in any of the holes in the puzzle, regardless of location.

For the most part, the THC fills the CB1 receptors. That's basically what gives that substance its psychoactive effect. Then, CBD typically fills in the CB2 receptors. And this is the reason it's effective at reducing joint pain, reducing gastrointestinal issues, as well as boosting your immune system.

Once all of these puzzle pieces are in place, the big picture is complete, and your body is in balance. Scientifically, this situation is referred to as homeostasis – the time when your body is not only properly maintained, but it's functioning maximum efficacy with the least amount of disease.

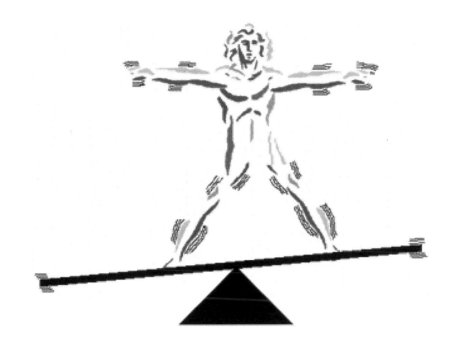

When your body is at homeostasis, it lets you think quicker, move faster, and respond more swiftly. As we said, this doesn't happen all the time, but when it does, you'll find athletes referring it to "the flow state", and others simply call it "the zone."

According to some, this flow state can also be attained with the precise combination of caffeine and cannabis. In this situation, the caffeine stimulates the brain, and the marijuana does the same thing to your body. This is essential when you're faced with making a quick decision which requires your complete focus and being completely "at the moment."

Exercise is necessary even when you utilize pot as part of your diet. But there is a silver lining. When I say "exercise," I don't necessarily mean spending time running on a treadmill or lifting weights or even working with those weight machines.

Instead, why not try some forms of exercise you may not have even considered before? Below are just a few of some remarkable activities you can perform to lose weight. Keep in mind that you'll be more likely to continue your exercise program if you find a friend to accompany you. At the very least, contact one of your friends and ask them to hold you accountable.

TRAIL RUNNING

Depending on the physical shape you're in, try trail running. If you can't do that, start off walking at a brisk pace. Find a bike path, a trail, or even a high school track field for this. Of course, you can go to the gym to hop on the treadmill, but you just may stay with the program that gets you outside, breathing fresh air, and enjoying the weather.

According to many researchers, and those who are already doing this, there is a strain of pot that would be the perfect pairing with this type of exercise – Panama Red, a sativa hybrid.

ROCK CLIMBING

This will be a tough outdoor activity if you're not living near any types of mountains. But don't give up hope. There are several excellent indoor rock climbing programs that can provide you with a nearly identical workout. This will be a good exercise if you're tired of going to the gym three times a week.

You'll probably find this activity the most entertaining (then it would seem less like a workout) if you gather up a few friends to go with you. Try pairing this activity with the Harlequin strain of marijuana or any other CBD strains that contain lower levels of THC.

TENNIS

Yes, indeed, tennis. If you've never considered learning the game, this would be a good time to give it some thought. While you can always find a way to practice on your own, all you need is a long, large wall with no windows; it would be more fun to get a group of friends together.

Some individuals try it at a later age and truly enjoy it. Chances are you'll never become a professional tennis player, but it's an excellent way to lose weight almost without knowing it. Keep in mind that the best type of marijuana to use with this activity is Headband and Trainwreck, both of which are sativa-dominant hybrids.

DANCING WITH THE ... FRIENDS

Dance. This is an excellent weight loss exercise. It doesn't matter what you do, Zumba, samba, ballroom, even pole dancing. Just get up and move. Don't worry what you look like or if anyone is watching; the idea is to get your body moving, for optimum weight loss and muscle strength. Play your favorite music and start moving your body.

Don't forget, if you are interested in dancing, you may want to think about taking classes. There are classes for all kinds of dancing, as well as private lessons. The strain of marijuana you may want to pair with this is either Durban Poison or Flo. Both are high-energy sativa.

Yoga

If you've already taken yoga classes or tried it on your own, then you already know the many benefits of yoga. Depending on the time of the year and the region of the country you live in, you may want to give an outdoor class a try. Or just grab a friend, a couple of yoga mats, and head for the nearest park.

Paired with Sour Diesel or Gorilla Glue, both sativa hybrids, you may never look at yoga the same way again.

CONCLUSION

The bottom line is that the only way you'll be successful in using marijuana as an integral part of your weight loss program is by customizing it to suit your needs. It's not a program that dictates how much you eat when you eat it, and what other foods you combine it with.

Eat healthy, exercise heartily, then smoke your choice of a strain of marijuana.

This book is a culmination of what I've learned trying to find my way in what can only be considered uncharted waters. A confluence of events has come together to experiment with it at this point in time.

The first is the widespread de-legalization of marijuana. In some states, pot has only been legalized for medicinal purposes. In others, recreational marijuana has also been decriminalized.

These actions have opened the floodgates to allow more serious scientific research to study the effects of this plant on not only weight loss, but your overall health. In the end, the two meet at a point where you have a unique opportunity to carefully and honestly evaluate your relationship to this potentially health-giving herb.

You'll find evidence of this as you sift through blogs about marijuana on the internet. Some individuals have discovered their "sweet spot" in smoking pot and losing weight. Others have reviewed their status and were faced with making some changes in their smoking habits as well as their exercise routine.

The following quotes and overall comments are given below to help you in your decision of whether this "diet plan" is right for you.

One blogger said, quite honestly, as he begins with an overarching powerful positive statement, "My ultimate conclusion so far: any experience can be much more superior and meaningful when I'm stoned."

That's a strong all-encompassing assertion. Then he continues and talks specifically about his weaving of marijuana use in his personalized exercise program. "I consume a high THC sativa [strain of marijuana] before each visit to the gym. I found high THC strains allow for relaxation in pre-workout stretching, better focus, and awareness of my body. . ."

But wait, his program doesn't end there. "Then I consumed CBD [strains] after the gym." He says this action helps him "wind down" from the intensity of his exercise.

Another blogger also admits to just beginning to see the best fit between her exercise and weight loss programs. She feels, so she says, like a "pioneer" in this area, and that's probably an accurate way to describe it.

She describes herself prior to exercising with marijuana as "unmotivated." She was unable to push past the necessary plateaus to jump to that next level. In fact, she was quite frank in saying that before her use of pot, she had "no desire to be a better version of herself."

After she decided on the strains that might help her motivation, she smoked marijuana both before, during, and after exercising. She was pleased with the results; a 45-pound weight loss which she has been able to keep off for two years.

But she has found that between the weight loss and the use of marijuana she has been able to rein in her previous anxiety and has improved her "overall quality of life tremendously."

While both of those individuals cited above sound as if they're using marijuana as an integral weight-loss tool, you also must understand that many individuals are making choices with this combination in ways that couldn't be called absolutely responsible.

By one writer's own admission, he would "get stoned out of his mind" before he put in his earbuds, loudly played a variety of music, and pushed his body, for the most part, past its physical limit. It's an interesting commentary on his actions and what he learned about his relationship with smoking and exercise.

If you're already a smoker and are even considering running or exercising at a full high, then read this. The author's done an excellent job of reviewing his actions and providing you with reasons for smoking and restraining your pot smoking while you exercise.

The article, though excellent, is too long to cite here in the detail it deserves.

http://flip.it/49HMSo

Lastly, since this is my first time writing such a book, I would appreciate if you find it in your heart to post a review, as it would the world to me.

Thank you so much!

Made in the USA
Columbia, SC
03 September 2024

41492493R00050